CBD OIL

Your Ultimate Guide to Choosing the Right CBD Oil to Alleviate Pain, Anxiety and Other Ailments

D1125439

Dr. London Barrett

Table of Contents

Chapter 1

CBD oil

Cannabidiol (CBD) is a chemical in the Cannabis sativa plant, additionally recognized as hashish or hemp. One unique structure of CBD is permitted as a drug in the U.S. for seizures.

Over eighty chemicals, regarded as cannabinoids, have been determined in the Cannabis sativa plant. Delta-9-tetrahydrocannabinol (THC) is the most well-known ingredient in cannabis. But CBD is received from hemp, a shape of the Cannabis sativa plant that solely consists of small quantities of THC. CBD looks to have results on some chemical substances in the brain, however these are exclusive than the consequences of THC.

A prescription shape of CBD is used for seizure disease (epilepsy). CBD is additionally used for anxiety, pain, a muscle sickness referred to as dystonia, Parkinson disease, Crohn disease, and many different conditions, however there is no appropriate scientific proof to assist these uses.

Laws surpassed in 2018 made it criminal to promote hemp and hemp merchandise in the US. But that would not suggest that all CBD merchandise made from hemp are legal. Since CBD is an accredited prescription drug, it cannot be legally blanketed in meals or dietary supplements. CBD can solely be protected in "cosmetic" products. But there are nonetheless CBD merchandise on the market that are labeled as dietary supplements. The quantity of CBD contained in these merchandise is no longer continually the identical as what is mentioned on the label. Potential aspect consequences of CBD products

Though CBD is commonly well-tolerated and is viewed safe, it might also motive damaging reactions in some people.

Side consequences referred to in research include:

diarrhea

changes in urge for food and weight

fatigue

Other aspect effects, which include odd liver feature take a look at results, drowsiness, sedation, and pneumonia, have been stated in childhood epilepsy studies. But these results may want to stem from CBD interacting with different medications, such as clobazam.

In fact, CBD interacts with numerous medications, consisting of ache medications, antidepressants, seizure medications, and diabetes medications. Before you strive CBD oil, talk about it with a healthcare expert to check security and keep away from doubtlessly damaging interactions.

Additionally, it's necessary to observe that the market is presently saturated with CBD products, many of which are low quality.

CBD is introduced to foods, beverages, dietary supplements, and physique care products, and these gadgets are regularly marketed as a way to enhance stress, pain, and sleep issues.

However, this does now not imply you ought to encompass any of these gadgets in your food regimen or health routine.

Although some proof suggests that CBD may additionally be

beneficial for positive components of health, dosing varies broadly in lookup studies. It's hard to decide what dose is most suitable for treating unique fitness needs.

What's more, many merchandise incorporate a combination of ingredients, no longer simply CBD. For example, dietary dietary supplements that include CBD plus a combination of natural elements may also now not be protected for everyone, as many herbs have the attainable to engage with many times prescribed medications.

Before you use a CBD product, discuss with a healthcare expert to talk about excellent dosing and any different questions you might also have.

If you do determine to use a CBD product, pick out one that has been third-party examined for exceptional and purity.

Chapter 2

What is CBD oil used for?

Supporters of CBD oil accept as true with it may also assist a range of medical conditions, which include refractory epilepsy, continual pain, depression, anxiousness and acne. However, in addition sturdy proof is required as an awful lot of the lookup is carried out on animal models.

A systematic assessment searching at the use of CBD for epilepsy concluded that there is inadequate proof to help the efficacy and long-term protection of the usage of it to deal with epilepsy. It does, however, advocate that, albeit in very low numbers, small day by day doses had been secure in a small crew of adults for a brief duration of time.

There are some pointers from animal research that CBD may also be recommended for osteoarthritis, via topical utility for infection or joint pain, however, it has been challenging to attribute the therapeutic advantages to CBT alone.

One find out about mentioned decreased ache and muscle

spasms in human beings with a couple of sclerosis.

Early proof searching into the use of CBD in the remedy of nervousness and despair has observed some thrilling outcomes – even though on very small samples. The first learn about assessed anxiousness hyperlinks with public speaking; it located a very precise dose of CBD (300mg) confirmed anti-anxiety effects. The 2nd find out about was once a stand-alone case document of one infant with post-traumatic stress disease (PTSD). It determined CBD oil helped the toddler safely decrease her anxiousness and enhance sleep.

CBD can also additionally have the doable to assist decrease acne; however, it is necessary to be aware that this lookup is nevertheless in its infancy.

What are some of the advantages of CBD?

Several research exhibit the advantages of pure CBD might also have wide-ranging wonderful effects, though. To apprehend these benefits, it's necessary to reflect on consideration on our body's endocannabinoid system, a complicated gadget of enzymes, neurotransmitters and receptors that performs an vital position in the improvement of our central anxious system. This device helps modify a range of functions, inclusive of pain, motor control, memory, appetite, infection and more. By in addition reading CBD's results in these precise areas, we might also higher apprehend how CBD influences a range of prerequisites and disorders.

Helps with neurological-related disorders

The FDA has accepted Epidiolex as a therapy for countless seizure disorders, along with two uncommon problems recognised as Duvet syndrome and Lennox-Gastaut syndrome. Several case research advocate CBD may also additionally be really helpful to sufferers who are resistant to anti-epileptic drugs. "With epilepsy, there's a threshold in your Genius that receives excitatory, and you go into a seizure.

Other research endorse CBD can also additionally be beneficial in managing signs of more than one sclerosis, Parkinson's sickness and Alzheimer's disease, as it has neuroprotective, anti-inflammatory properties. More research are needed, however, as many propose that it's no longer simply CBD alone, however a mixture of CBD and different cannabinoids, that may also assist decrease many of these symptoms.

It might also aid with ache relief

By interacting with neurotransmitters in your central fearful system, CBD should doubtlessly relieve ache associated to inflammation, arthritis and nerve injury (peripheral neuropathy). In one four-week trial, humans who had nerve harm in the decrease 1/2 of their physique mentioned a big discount of intense, sharp ache after the usage of a topical CBD oil.

"All of our unique anti-pain tablets have an effect on some area of our ache system, whether or not it's Tylenol®, Aspirin®, morphine or opioids. "No one needs to be addicted to opioids, so if there's a cannabinoid you can take that's now not addictive however can repress the pain, that would be the Holy Grail with persistent pain."

What is the chance of taking cannabinoid oil?

While extensively circulated communications recommend cannabinoid oils are protected and do now not intrude with different medication, in reality, investigations have proven actual interference with any anti-epileptic capsules metabolised (broken down) by way of the liver. We have additionally had journey of hashish oils interfering with sturdy ache killers. Most automatically used medicinal drugs have now not but been examined in aggregate with cannabinoids. There is a possible hazard for interplay with in many instances prescribed medicinal drugs for different conditions.

Known side-effects of cannabinoids decided from scientific trials encompass sedation, urge for food suppression, diarrhoea, dizziness and odd liver function.

We have no actual statistics on the side-effect profile of cannabinoid oils, particularly in younger children, who may also be extraordinarily touchy to small doses. In addition, younger youngsters are regularly unable to precisely describe damaging consequences that means toxicity can also be below reported.

Chapter 3

What CBD Oil Can Interact With

CBD oil can engage with medications, along with many that are used to treat epilepsy. One of the motives for this has to do with how your physique breaks down (metabolizes) drugs.

Cytochrome P450 (CYP450) is an enzyme your physique makes use of to wreck down some drugs. CBD oil can block CYP450. That ability that taking CBD oil with these pills should make them have a enhanced impact than you want or make them no longer work at all.

Drugs that may want to probably have interaction with CBD include:

Anti-arrhythmia tablets like quinidine

Anticonvulsants like Tegretol (carbamazepine) and Trileptal (oxcarbazepine)

Antifungal pills like Nizoral (ketoconazole) and Vfend (voriconazole)

Antipsychotic capsules like Orap (pimozide)

Atypical antidepressants like Remeron (mirtazapine)

Benzodiazepine sedatives like Klonopin (clonazepam) and Halcion (triazolam)

Immune-suppressive pills like Sandimmune (cyclosporine)

Macrolide antibiotics like clarithromycin and telithromycin

Migraine medication like Ergomar (ergotamine)

Opioid painkillers like Duragesic (fentanyl) and alfentanil

Rifampin-based capsules used to deal with tuberculosis

How to use CBD

There are a number approaches of the use of CBD oil. These are now not the identical as the use of or smoking total cannabis.

If a health practitioner prescribes CBD for epilepsy, it is necessary to comply with their instructions.

Ways of the usage of CBD merchandise include:

- mixing them into meals or drink

- taking them with a pipette or dropper

- swallowing capsules

- massaging a paste into the skin

- spraying it below the tongue

Recommended dosages range between men and women and rely on elements such as:

body weight

the attention of the product

the cause for the usage of CBD

Special Precautions and Warnings

Pregnancy and breast-feeding: It might also be hazardous to take CBD if you are pregnant or breast feeding. CBD merchandise can be contaminated with different elements that may additionally be damaging to the fetus or infant. Stay on the protected aspect and keep away from use.

Children: It is perchance protected for youth to take a precise prescription CBD product (Epidiolex) by means of mouth in doses up to 25 mg/kg daily. This product is accepted for use in young people with sure stipulations who are at least 1 12 months old. It is not clear if different CBD merchandise are protected in children.

Liver disease: People with liver sickness may also want to use decrease doses of CBD.

Parkinson disease: Some early lookup suggests that taking excessive doses of CBD would possibly make muscle motion and tremors worse in some humans with Parkinson disease.

What's a Safe Dosage of CBD Oil?

There are no tips for use, nor is there a "correct" dose of CBD oil. That said, the common dose vary is from 5 mg to 25 mg.

Available types include:

- Tinctures (CBD oil blended with a base oil)

- Capsules

- Gummies

- Sprays

Which you select generally comes down to your desire and what you hope to get in phrases of effects. For example, inserting the oil underneath your tongue can produce consequences extra shortly than swallowing a pill that wants to be digested.

Each product works a bit differently, relying on the form, so it is essential to observe the furnished directions.

How to Calculate a CBD Dose

Sprays, gummies, and pills are effortless to use due to the fact their doses are pre-measured.

Tinctures are a bit extra challenging. Most oils come in

30-milliliter (mL) bottles and consist of a dropper cap to assist you measure.

But some tinctures have concentrations of 1,500 mg per 30 mL, whilst others have 3,000 mg per mL or more. That capacity figuring out the precise quantity of CBD per milliliter of oil requires a little math.

To decide an actual dose of CBD, understand that every drop of oil equals 0.05 mL of fluid. This ability that a 30-mL bottle of CBD oil will have about 600 drops in it.

If the awareness of the tincture is 1,500 mg per mL, one drop would have 2.5 mg of CBD in it (1,500 mg ÷ 600 drops = 2.5 mg).

Chapter 4

How can CBD be taken?

CBD comes in many forms, which includes oils, extracts, capsules, patches, vapes, and topical preparations for use on skin. If you're hoping to decrease infection and relieve muscle and joint pain, a topical CBD-infused oil, lotion or cream – or even a tub bomb -- may additionally be the fine option. Alternatively, a CBC patch or a tincture or spray designed to be positioned underneath the tongue lets in CBD to at once enter the bloodstream.

Outside of the US, the prescription drug Sativex, which makes use of CBD as an lively ingredient, is accredited for muscle spasticity related with a couple of sclerosis and for most cancers pain. Within the US, Epidiolex is accepted for sure sorts of epilepsy and tuberous sclerosis.

The bottom line on cannabidiol

Some CBD producers have come below authorities scrutiny for wild, indefensible claims, such that CBD is a cure-all for most cancers or COVID-19, which it is not. We want greater lookup however CBD may also show to be a helpful, quite non-toxic alternative for managing anxiety, insomnia, and persistent pain. Without adequate tremendous proof in human studies, we can't pinpoint high-quality doses, and due to the fact CBD presently is commonly handy as an unregulated supplement, it's challenging to understand precisely what you are getting.

If you figure out to attempt CBD, make positive you are getting it from a official source. And speak with your health practitioner to make certain that

it won't have an effect on any
different drug treatments you
take.

THE END

Made in the USA
Middletown, DE
28 April 2023